COPYR

CW01475584

Copyright © Precious Anusiem

ABOUT AUTHOR

Precious Anusiem, is a multi-talented tech entrepreneur, programmer, and writer whose passion for technology, business, and writing has been a driving force since childhood. Precious has always been a visionary, constantly seeking out innovative ways to make life easier and better for humanity.

From a young age, Precious demonstrated a remarkable aptitude for learning and a keen ability to think outside the box. This relentless curiosity and drive have propelled her to master an impressive array of computer-based skills and technologies. Her expertise spans across writing, programming, analysis, content creation, cybersecurity, AI engineering and many others.

Precious embodies the spirit of continuous learning and self-improvement. Her unique approach, experience in the medical field and dedication to excellence set her apart.

OTHER TOP BOOKS

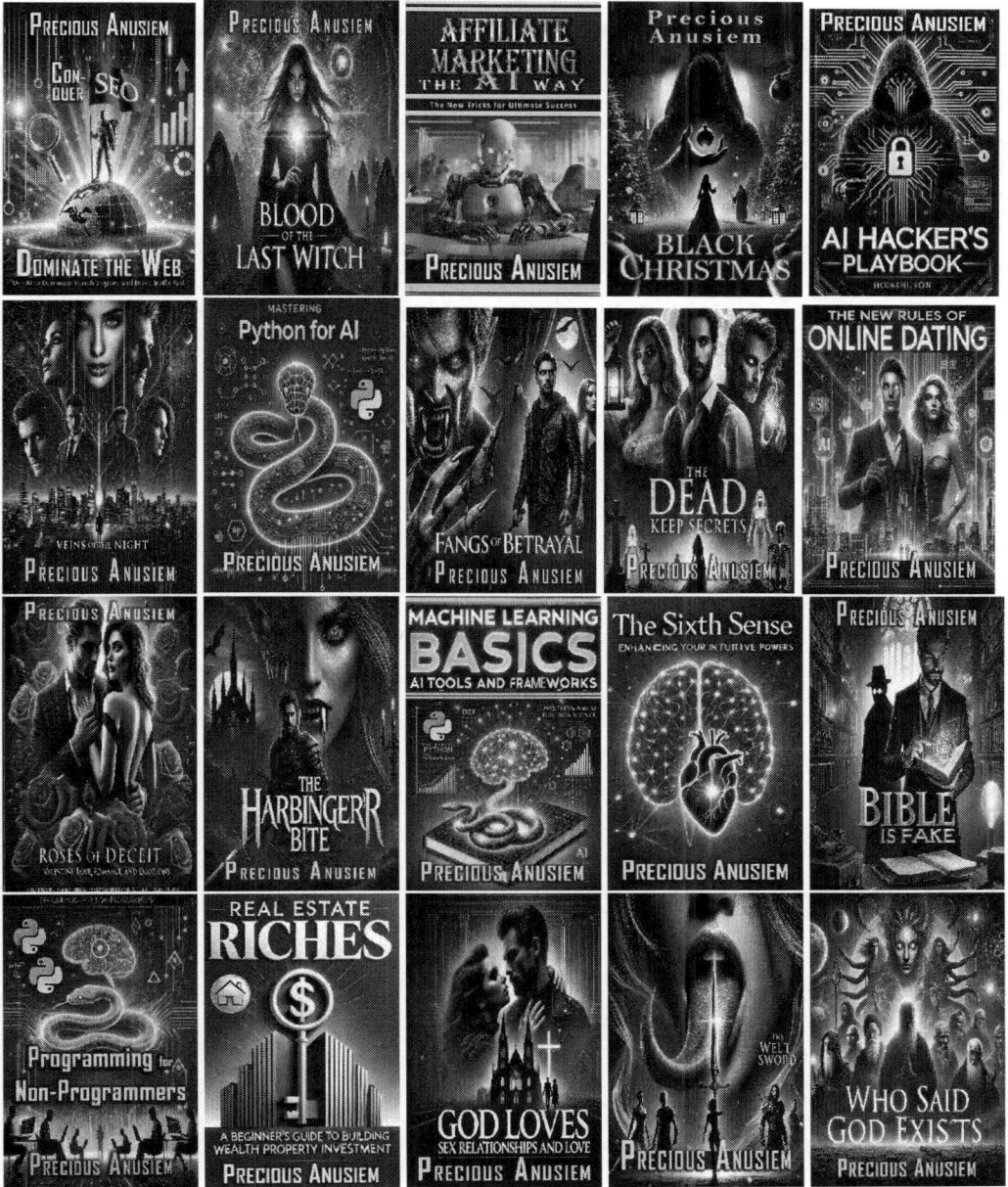

Precious Anusiem — CONQUER SEO — DOMINATE THE WEB

Precious Anusiem — BLOOD OF THE LAST WITCH

AFFILIATE MARKETING THE AI WAY — The New Tricks for Ultimate Success — Precious Anusiem

Precious Anusiem — BLACK CHRISTMAS

Precious Anusiem — AI HACKER'S PLAYBOOK

VEINS OF THE NIGHT — Precious Anusiem

MASTERING Python for AI — Precious Anusiem

FANGS OF BETRAYAL — Precious Anusiem

THE DEAD KEEP SECRETS — Precious Anusiem

THE NEW RULES OF ONLINE DATING — Precious Anusiem

ROSES OF DECEIT — Precious Anusiem

THE HARBINGER'R BITE — Precious Anusiem

MACHINE LEARNING BASICS — AI TOOLS AND FRAMEWORKS — Precious Anusiem

The Sixth Sense — ENHANCING YOUR INTUITIVE POWERS — Precious Anusiem

Precious Anusiem — BIBLE IS FAKE

Programming for Non-Programmers — Precious Anusiem

REAL ESTATE RICHES — A BEGINNER'S GUIDE TO BUILDING WEALTH PROPERTY INVESTMENT — Precious Anusiem

GOD LOVES SEX RELATIONSHIPS AND LOVE — Precious Anusiem

THE WELT SWORD — Precious Anusiem

WHO SAID GOD EXISTS — Precious Anusiem

Visit "https://www.amazon.com/author/preciousanusiem" to access all books both **fiction** and **non-fiction** books.

Introduction:

Why Fitness Matters When You Have Diabetes

Living with diabetes isn't a walk in the park. It's a daily grind of pricking your finger, counting carbs, and trying to figure out how that slice of pizza you ate two hours ago is going to mess with your blood sugar. It's exhausting, frustrating, and sometimes downright overwhelming. But here's the thing: you're not powerless. In fact, one of the most powerful tools you have to manage diabetes is something you might not even realize—exercise.

Now, I know what you're thinking. "Exercise? Really? I can barely find time to brush my teeth in the morning, let alone hit the gym." Trust me, I get it. Life is busy, and when you're juggling work, family, and everything else, adding one more thing to your plate can feel impossible. But here's the kicker—exercise doesn't have to be complicated, time-consuming, or even sweaty (unless you want it to be). It can be as simple as taking a walk around your neighborhood or doing a few stretches while you're watching TV.

The truth is, exercise is one of the most effective ways to manage blood sugar levels, improve insulin sensitivity, and boost your overall health. And the best part? You don't have to run a marathon or lift heavy weights to see results. Small, consistent changes can make a huge difference.

The Science Behind Exercise and Diabetes

Let's get a little nerdy for a second. When you exercise, your muscles use glucose (sugar) for energy. This helps lower your blood sugar levels, both during and after your workout. Over time, regular physical activity can also improve your body's ability to use insulin, which is crucial for managing diabetes.

But it's not just about blood sugar. Exercise has a ton of other benefits, too. It can help you lose weight, reduce stress, improve your heart health, and even boost your mood. And when you're living with diabetes, anything that makes you feel better is worth trying.

Breaking Down the Myths

Before we dive into the nitty-gritty, let's clear up some common misconceptions about exercise and diabetes.

1. Myth: You need to exercise for hours to see results.

Truth: Even 10 minutes of physical activity can make a difference. The key is consistency.

2. Myth: Only intense workouts count.

Truth: Low-impact activities like walking, swimming, and yoga are just as effective (and often safer) for people with diabetes.

3. Myth: Exercise is dangerous if you have diabetes.

Truth: As long as you take the right precautions (like checking your blood sugar before and after exercise), physical activity is safe and beneficial.

The Emotional Side of Diabetes

Let's talk about something that doesn't get enough attention—the emotional toll of living with diabetes. It's not just about managing numbers; it's about dealing with the constant stress, anxiety, and frustration that come with the condition.

I've worked with countless individuals who've told me they feel like they're fighting a losing battle. They're tired of feeling like their body is working against them, and they're scared of what the future might hold. But here's the thing—exercise can be a game-changer, not just physically, but emotionally, too.

When you exercise, your body releases endorphins, which are natural mood boosters. It's like getting a dose of happiness without the side effects. Plus, the sense of accomplishment you feel after completing a workout can be incredibly empowering.

Why This Book is Different

There are a ton of books out there about diabetes and exercise, so why should you read this one? Here's the deal—this book isn't just about giving you a list of exercises to do. It's about empowering you to take control of your health in a way that works for you.

I've spent years working with people with diabetes, and I've seen firsthand how overwhelming it can be to navigate all the conflicting advice out there. That's why this book is designed to be practical, realistic, and, most importantly, doable.

You won't find any complicated routines or unrealistic expectations here. Instead, you'll get simple, actionable advice that you can start using today. Whether you're a complete beginner or someone who's been exercising for years, this book has something for you.

What You'll Learn

Here's a sneak peek at what you'll find in this book:

- The Best Exercises for Managing Blood Sugar: From walking to strength training, we'll cover the most effective workouts for people with diabetes.

- How to Stay Safe While Exercising: Tips for avoiding low blood sugar, staying hydrated, and preventing injuries.

- Creating a Personalized Fitness Plan: Step-by-step guidance on how to build a routine that fits your lifestyle and goals.

- Overcoming Common Challenges: Strategies for staying motivated, dealing with setbacks, and making exercise a habit.

- The Role of Nutrition: How to fuel your workouts and manage your blood sugar through smart food choices.

A Word of Encouragement

If you're feeling overwhelmed or unsure about where to start, that's okay. You're not alone. The fact that you're reading this book means you're already taking a step in the right direction.

Chapter 1

Understanding Diabetes and Exercise

If you're living with diabetes, you already know it's a condition where your body struggles to manage blood sugar (glucose) levels. But what you might not realize is how much exercise can impact those levels—for the better. Exercise isn't just about losing weight or building muscle (though those are great perks). For people with diabetes, it's a powerful tool to help regulate blood sugar, improve insulin sensitivity, and boost overall health.

But before we dive into the "how," let's talk about the "why." Why does exercise work so well for managing diabetes? And how can you use it to your advantage without feeling overwhelmed or risking your health? That's what this chapter is all about.

How Exercise Affects Blood Sugar

When you exercise, your muscles need energy to keep moving. That energy comes from glucose, which is stored in your muscles and liver. As you work out, your body pulls glucose from your bloodstream to fuel your muscles. This process helps lower your blood sugar levels, both during and after your workout.

But here's the kicker—exercise doesn't just help in the short term. Over time, regular physical activity can improve your body's ability to use insulin, the hormone that helps regulate blood sugar. This is especially important for people with Type 2 diabetes, where insulin resistance is a common issue.

The Benefits of Exercise for Diabetes

Let's break it down. Here's why exercise is a game-changer for people with diabetes:

1. Lowers Blood Sugar Levels: As mentioned, exercise helps your muscles use glucose for energy, which can lower your blood sugar levels.

2. Improves Insulin Sensitivity: Regular physical activity makes your body more responsive to insulin, which can help manage Type 2 diabetes.

3. Aids in Weight Management: Maintaining a healthy weight is crucial for managing diabetes, and exercise is a key part of that.

4. Reduces Risk of Complications: Exercise can lower your risk of heart disease, nerve damage, and other diabetes-related complications.

5. Boosts Mental Health: Living with diabetes can be stressful, and exercise is a natural mood booster.

Even if you don't see immediate changes in your blood sugar levels, don't get discouraged. The benefits of exercise build up over time, so consistency is key.

Types of Exercise and Their Impact

Not all exercises are created equal, especially when it comes to managing diabetes. Here's a breakdown of the most effective types:

1. Aerobic Exercise

Aerobic exercise, also known as cardio, is any activity that gets your heart rate up. Think walking, cycling, swimming, or dancing. These exercises are great for lowering blood sugar levels because they increase your body's demand for glucose.

- Walking: It's simple, accessible, and effective. Aim for 30 minutes a day, five days a week.

- Cycling: Whether it's on a stationary bike or outdoors, cycling is a low-impact way to get your heart pumping.

- Swimming: Perfect for those with joint issues, swimming provides a full-body workout without putting stress on your joints.

2. Strength Training

Strength training, also known as resistance training, involves using weights, resistance bands, or your own body weight to build muscle. This type of exercise is especially beneficial for people with diabetes because muscle tissue burns more glucose than fat tissue.

- Bodyweight Exercises: Squats, lunges, and push-ups are great for beginners.

- Resistance Bands: These portable tools are perfect for adding resistance to your workouts without needing heavy weights.

- Weight Lifting: If you're comfortable, incorporate dumbbells or kettlebells into your routine.

Start with lighter weights and focus on proper form. It's better to do fewer reps correctly than to risk injury.

3. Flexibility and Balance Exercises

While these exercises don't directly lower blood sugar, they're essential for overall health and injury prevention.

- Yoga: Improves flexibility, reduces stress, and can even help with blood sugar control.
- Tai Chi: This gentle form of exercise is great for balance and relaxation.

How to Get Started

If you're new to exercise, the idea of starting a fitness routine can feel overwhelming. But here's the thing—you don't have to run a marathon or lift heavy weights to see results. Small, consistent changes can make a huge difference.

1. Start Slow: Begin with low-impact activities like walking or gentle yoga. Gradually increase intensity as your fitness improves.

2. Set Realistic Goals: Aim for 10-15 minutes of exercise a day to start. As you build stamina, you can increase the duration and intensity.

3. Find Activities You Enjoy: Exercise doesn't have to be a chore. Whether it's dancing, hiking, or playing with your kids, find something that makes you happy.

4. Track Your Progress: Keep a journal of your workouts and blood sugar levels to see how your body responds.

Don't be afraid to ask for help. A certified personal trainer or diabetes educator can help you create a safe and effective exercise plan.

Safety Tips for Exercising with Diabetes

Exercise is generally safe for people with diabetes, but there are a few precautions you should take:

1. Check Your Blood Sugar: Always check your blood sugar before and after exercise, especially if you're new to working out.

2. Stay Hydrated: Dehydration can affect blood sugar levels, so drink plenty of water before, during, and after exercise.

3. Have a Snack Handy: Keep a fast-acting carbohydrate (like glucose tablets or fruit juice) nearby in case your blood sugar drops too low.

4. Listen to Your Body: If you feel dizzy, fatigued, or unwell, stop exercising and check your blood sugar.

The Emotional Benefits of Exercise

Let's not forget the mental and emotional side of things. Living with diabetes can be stressful, and exercise is a natural stress reliever. When you exercise, your body releases endorphins, which are natural mood boosters. It's like getting a dose of happiness without the side effects.

Plus, the sense of accomplishment you feel after completing a workout can be incredibly empowering. It's a reminder that you're in control of your health, even when it feels like your body is working against you.

Chapter 2

Getting Started—Safety First

Starting a fitness routine can feel like stepping into the unknown, especially when you're managing diabetes. You might be wondering, "What if my blood sugar drops too low? What if I hurt myself? What if I just can't stick with it?" These are valid concerns, and they're exactly why we're diving into this chapter.

The truth is, exercise is one of the best things you can do for your health, but it's not without its risks. That's why safety comes first. Whether you're a complete beginner or someone who's been active for years, taking the right precautions can make all the difference.

Why Safety Matters

When you have diabetes, your body doesn't regulate blood sugar the way it should. This means you need to be extra careful when you're exercising, as physical activity can cause your blood sugar levels to fluctuate.

For example, if your blood sugar is too low before you start exercising, you could be at risk of hypoglycemia (low blood sugar). On the flip side, if your blood sugar is too high, you might be at risk of hyperglycemia (high blood sugar). Both scenarios can be dangerous if not managed properly.

But don't let this scare you off. With the right precautions, you can exercise safely and effectively. It's all about being prepared and listening to your body.

Step 1: Talk to Your Doctor

Before you lace up those sneakers, the first thing you need to do is talk to your healthcare provider. I know, I know—it's not the most exciting step, but it's crucial. Your doctor can help you determine what types of exercise are safe for you, how to monitor your blood sugar, and whether you need to adjust your medications.

Step 2: Start Slow

If you're new to exercise, the key is to start slow. You don't have to run a 5K or lift heavy weights on day one. In fact, jumping into intense workouts too quickly can do more harm than good.

Here's how to ease into it:

1. Begin with Low-Impact Activities: Walking, swimming, and gentle yoga are great options for beginners.

2. Set Realistic Goals: Aim for 10-15 minutes of exercise a day to start. As you build stamina, you can increase the duration and intensity.

3. Listen to Your Body: If something doesn't feel right, stop and take a break. It's better to be cautious than to risk injury.

Try exercising after meals when your blood sugar levels are higher. This can help prevent lows and give you more energy for your workout.

Step 3: Monitor Your Blood Sugar

Checking your blood sugar before, during, and after exercise is one of the most important things you can do to stay safe. Here's why:

- Before Exercise: This helps you determine whether it's safe to work out. If your blood sugar is too low (below 100 mg/dL), have a small snack before starting. If it's too high (above 250 mg/dL), you may need to wait until it comes down.

- During Exercise: If you're doing a longer workout, check your blood sugar every 30 minutes to make sure it's stable.

- After Exercise: Exercise can lower your blood sugar for several hours after you finish, so it's important to check your levels and have a snack if needed.

Step 4: Stay Hydrated

Dehydration can affect your blood sugar levels and make it harder for your body to regulate temperature during exercise. That's why it's important to drink plenty of water before, during, and after your workout.

Here are some tips to stay hydrated:

- Drink Water Before You're Thirsty: Thirst is a sign that you're already dehydrated, so sip water throughout the day.
- Avoid Sugary Drinks: Stick to water or sugar-free beverages to avoid blood sugar spikes.
- Carry a Water Bottle: Keep a reusable water bottle with you so you can stay hydrated on the go.

If you're doing a long or intense workout, consider a sports drink with electrolytes to replace what you lose through sweat. Just make sure it's low in sugar.

Step 5: Have a Snack Handy

Even if you check your blood sugar before exercising, it's always a good idea to have a fast-acting carbohydrate nearby in case your levels drop too low.

Some good options include:

- Glucose Tablets: These are quick and easy to carry.

- Fruit Juice: A small box of juice can help raise your blood sugar quickly.

- Candy: Hard candies or gummies are portable and effective.

Step 6: Dress for Success

What you wear during exercise might not seem like a big deal, but it can make a difference, especially if you have diabetes.

- Wear Comfortable Shoes: Proper footwear is essential to prevent blisters, sores, and other foot issues.

- Choose Breathable Fabrics: Moisture-wicking clothing can help keep you cool and dry during your workout.

- Protect Your Feet: If you have neuropathy (nerve damage), make sure to check your feet for cuts or sores after exercising.

Invest in a good pair of shoes that fit well and provide support. Your feet will thank you.

Step 7: Listen to Your Body

At the end of the day, the most important thing is to listen to your body. If something doesn't feel right, stop and take a break. It's better to be cautious than to risk injury or a blood sugar emergency.

Here are some signs to watch out for:

- Dizziness or Lightheadedness: This could be a sign of low blood sugar.

- Chest Pain or Shortness of Breath: Stop exercising and seek medical attention immediately.

- Extreme Fatigue: If you're feeling unusually tired, it might be time to call it a day.

Chapter 3

The Best Exercises for Managing Blood Sugar

Alright, let's get into the good stuff—the exercises that can help you manage your blood sugar levels effectively. If you've made it this far, you already know that exercise is a powerful tool for managing diabetes. But what you might not know is which exercises work best and how to incorporate them into your routine without feeling overwhelmed.

Why Exercise Choices Matter

Not all exercises are created equal, especially when it comes to managing diabetes. Some are better at lowering blood sugar in the short term, while others help improve insulin sensitivity over time. The key is to find a balance that works for you.

The best exercise routine is one you'll actually stick with. It doesn't matter how effective an exercise is if you hate doing it. So, while we'll cover the most scientifically backed exercises for managing blood sugar, we'll also talk about how to make them enjoyable and sustainable.

Aerobic Exercise: The Blood Sugar Regulator

Aerobic exercise, also known as cardio, is any activity that gets your heart rate up and keeps it there for a sustained period. Think walking, cycling, swimming, or dancing. These exercises are fantastic for lowering blood sugar levels because they increase your body's demand for glucose.

1. Walking

Let's start with the simplest and most accessible form of aerobic exercise—walking. You don't need any special equipment, and you can do it almost anywhere.

- How to Get Started: Start with a 10-minute walk around your neighborhood. Gradually increase the duration and pace as your fitness improves.

- Why It Works: Walking helps your muscles use glucose for energy, which can lower your blood sugar levels. Plus, it's easy on the joints.

2. Cycling

Cycling is another great option, whether you prefer a stationary bike or hitting the trails.

- How to Get Started: If you're new to cycling, start with 10-15 minutes on a stationary bike. Gradually increase the duration and resistance as you build stamina.

- Why It Works: Cycling is a low-impact exercise that gets your heart pumping and helps your body use glucose more efficiently.

If you're cycling outdoors, make sure to wear a helmet and choose safe, well-lit routes.

3. Swimming

Swimming is perfect for those with joint issues or anyone looking for a full-body workout.

- How to Get Started: Begin with 10-15 minutes of gentle swimming or water aerobics. Gradually increase the duration and intensity as you get more comfortable.

- Why It Works: Swimming provides a cardiovascular workout without putting stress on your joints, making it ideal for people with diabetes.

Strength Training: Building Muscle, Lowering Blood Sugar

Strength training, also known as resistance training, involves using weights, resistance bands, or your own body weight to build muscle. This type of exercise is especially beneficial for people with diabetes because muscle tissue burns more glucose than fat tissue.

1. Bodyweight Exercises

If you're new to strength training, bodyweight exercises are a great place to start.

- Examples: Squats, lunges, push-ups, and planks.
- How to Get Started: Begin with 1-2 sets of 8-10 repetitions for each exercise. Focus on proper form and gradually increase the number of sets and reps as you get stronger.

- Why It Works: Bodyweight exercises help build muscle, which can improve insulin sensitivity over time.

If you're not sure how to do an exercise correctly, consider working with a personal trainer or watching instructional videos online.

2. Resistance Bands

Resistance bands are portable, affordable, and versatile, making them a great option for strength training.

- Examples: Band pull-aparts, bicep curls, and leg presses.
- How to Get Started: Choose a band with the right level of resistance for your fitness level. Start with 1-2 sets of 8-10 repetitions for each exercise.

- Why It Works: Resistance bands provide a low-impact way to build muscle and improve insulin sensitivity.

3. Weight Lifting

If you're comfortable with weights, incorporating dumbbells or kettlebells into your routine can take your strength training to the next level.

- Examples: Dumbbell squats, kettlebell swings, and bench presses.

- How to Get Started: Begin with lighter weights and focus on proper form. Gradually increase the weight as you get stronger.

- Why It Works: Weight lifting builds muscle mass, which can help improve long-term blood sugar control.

Always warm up before lifting weights and cool down afterward to prevent injury.

Flexibility and Balance Exercises: The Unsung Heroes

While flexibility and balance exercises don't directly lower blood sugar, they're essential for overall health and injury prevention.

1. Yoga

Yoga combines stretching, strength, and mindfulness, making it a great option for people with diabetes.

- How to Get Started: Look for beginner-friendly yoga classes online or at a local studio. Start with 10-15 minutes a day and gradually increase the duration.

- Why It Works: Yoga improves flexibility, reduces stress, and can even help with blood sugar control.

2. Tai Chi

Tai Chi is a gentle form of exercise that focuses on slow, controlled movements and deep breathing.

- How to Get Started: Look for beginner Tai Chi classes online or in your community. Start with 10-15 minutes a day and gradually increase the duration.

- Why It Works: Tai Chi improves balance, reduces stress, and can help with blood sugar control.

Tai Chi is especially beneficial for older adults or anyone with balance issues.

Putting It All Together

The best exercise routine is one that includes a mix of aerobic, strength, and flexibility exercises. Here's a sample weekly plan to get you started:

- Monday: 30-minute walk

- Tuesday: Bodyweight exercises (squats, lunges, push-ups)

- Wednesday: Yoga or Tai Chi

- Thursday: 30-minute swim or cycle

- Friday: Resistance band workout

- Saturday: 30-minute walk

- Sunday: Rest or gentle stretching

Chapter 4

Creating Your Personalized Fitness Plan

Starting a fitness routine can feel like trying to solve a Rubik's Cube blindfolded—confusing, frustrating, and maybe even a little intimidating. But here's the thing: it doesn't have to be that way. With the right plan, you can make exercise a seamless part of your life, even when you're managing diabetes.

Step 1: Define Your Goals

Before you start any fitness plan, it's important to know what you're working toward. Your goals will shape everything from the types of exercises you do to how often you do them.

Here are some common goals for people with diabetes:

- Lowering Blood Sugar Levels: Regular exercise can help stabilize your blood sugar and improve insulin sensitivity.

- Losing Weight: Maintaining a healthy weight is crucial for managing diabetes and reducing the risk of complications.

- Improving Energy Levels: Exercise can boost your stamina and help you feel more energized throughout the day.

- Reducing Stress: Physical activity is a natural stress reliever, which is especially important when you're managing a chronic condition.

Step 2: Assess Your Current Fitness Level

Let's be honest—you can't create a realistic fitness plan if you don't know where you're starting from. Assessing your current fitness level will help you determine what types of exercises are appropriate and how to progress safely.

Here's how to do it:

1. Cardiovascular Fitness: How long can you walk, jog, or cycle without feeling out of breath?

2. Strength: Can you do basic bodyweight exercises like squats or push-ups? If so, how many?

3. Flexibility: Can you touch your toes or perform simple stretches without discomfort?

4. Balance: Can you stand on one leg for 30 seconds without losing your balance?

Don't compare yourself to others. This is about understanding your starting point so you can make progress at your own pace.

Step 3: Choose Activities You Enjoy

Here's a hard truth: if you hate running, you're not going to stick with a running routine. The key to long-term success is choosing activities you actually enjoy.

Here are some ideas to get you started:

- If You Love the Outdoors: Try hiking, cycling, or gardening.

- If You Prefer Group Activities: Join a dance class, water aerobics, or a sports league.

- If You're a Homebody: Try yoga, bodyweight exercises, or online workout videos.

Step 4: Create a Balanced Routine

A well-rounded fitness plan includes a mix of aerobic, strength, flexibility, and balance exercises. Here's how to structure your week:

Aerobic Exercise

Aim for at least 150 minutes of moderate-intensity aerobic exercise per week. This could include:

- Walking: 30 minutes, 5 days a week.

- Cycling: 20-30 minutes, 3-4 days a week.

- Swimming: 20-30 minutes, 2-3 days a week.

Strength Training

Incorporate strength training exercises at least 2-3 days a week. This could include:

- Bodyweight Exercises: Squats, lunges, push-ups.

- Resistance Bands: Band pull-aparts, bicep curls.

- Weight Lifting: Dumbbell squats, kettlebell swings.

Flexibility and Balance

Include flexibility and balance exercises 2-3 days a week. This could include:

- Yoga: 10-15 minutes of gentle stretching.
- Tai Chi: 10-15 minutes of slow, controlled movements.

Don't feel like you have to do everything at once. Start with one or two types of exercise and gradually add more as you get comfortable.

Step 5: Schedule Your Workouts

If you don't schedule your workouts, they probably won't happen. Life gets busy, and it's easy to push exercise to the bottom of your to-do list.

Here's how to make it work:

1. Choose a Time That Works for You: Whether it's first thing in the morning, during your lunch break, or after dinner, find a time that fits your schedule.

2. Start Small: If you're new to exercise, start with 10-15 minutes a day and gradually increase the duration.

3. Be Consistent: Try to exercise at the same time each day to build a habit.

Step 6: Track Your Progress

Tracking your progress is a great way to stay motivated and see how far you've come. Here's how to do it:

1. Keep a Workout Journal: Write down what you did, how long you did it, and how you felt.

2. Monitor Your Blood Sugar: Check your levels before and after exercise to see how your body responds.

3. Celebrate Small Wins: Did you walk an extra 5 minutes today? That's a win!

Use a fitness app or wearable device to track your steps, heart rate, and other metrics.

Step 7: Adjust as Needed

Your fitness plan isn't set in stone. As you get stronger and more confident, you can adjust your routine to keep challenging yourself.

Here's how to do it:

1. Increase Intensity: Add more resistance, speed, or duration to your workouts.

2. Try New Activities: Mix things up to keep your routine interesting.

3. Listen to Your Body: If something doesn't feel right, don't be afraid to mod

Chapter 5

Overcoming Common Challenges

Starting and sticking to a fitness routine isn't always a walk in the park. Life gets in the way. Motivation wanes. Blood sugar levels fluctuate. And sometimes, it feels like the universe is conspiring against you. But here's the thing: every challenge you face is an opportunity to grow stronger, both physically and mentally.

Challenge 1: Lack of Time

"I don't have time to exercise." Sound familiar? It's one of the most common excuses out there, and honestly, it's a valid one. Between work, family, and everything else on your plate, finding time to work out can feel impossible.

But here's the thing: you don't need hours to make a difference. Even 10 minutes of exercise can have a positive impact on your blood sugar levels and overall health.

Strategies to Overcome Time Constraints

1. Break It Up: Instead of trying to do one long workout, break it into smaller chunks. For example, three 10-minute walks throughout the day are just as effective as one 30-minute walk.

2. Multitask: Combine exercise with other activities. Walk while you're on the phone, do squats while you're brushing your teeth, or stretch while you're watching TV.

3. Schedule It: Treat exercise like an appointment. Block off time in your calendar and stick to it.

Challenge 2: Low Motivation

Some days, you just don't feel like working out. And that's okay. Motivation comes and goes, but discipline and habits can keep you going even when you're not feeling it.

Strategies to Boost Motivation

1. Find Your Why: Remind yourself why you started. Is it to feel better? To have more energy? To spend more time with your loved ones? Write it down and keep it somewhere visible.

2. Set Small Goals: Instead of focusing on the big picture, set small, achievable goals. For example, aim to walk 10 minutes today or do five push-ups.

3. Get an Accountability Partner: Find a friend, family member, or workout buddy to keep you on track.

Create a workout playlist with your favorite songs. Music can be a powerful motivator.

Challenge 3: Fear of Low Blood Sugar

For many people with diabetes, the fear of low blood sugar (hypoglycemia) is a major barrier to exercise. And it's a valid concern—low blood sugar can be dangerous if not managed properly.

Strategies to Prevent Low Blood Sugar

1. Check Your Levels: Always check your blood sugar before and after exercise. If it's too low (below 100 mg/dL), have a small snack before starting.

2. Carry Fast-Acting Carbs: Keep glucose tablets, fruit juice, or candy nearby in case your blood sugar drops during your workout.

3. Adjust Your Medications: Talk to your doctor about adjusting your insulin or other medications if you're exercising regularly.

Challenge 4: Boredom

Let's be honest—doing the same workout over and over can get boring. And when you're bored, it's easy to lose motivation.

Strategies to Beat Boredom

1. Mix It Up: Try new activities to keep things interesting. If you usually walk, try cycling or swimming instead.

2. Join a Class: Group fitness classes can be a fun way to stay motivated and meet new people.

3. Set Challenges: Challenge yourself to try something new, like a 5K run or a yoga pose you've never done before.

Use apps or online videos to try new workouts from the comfort of your home.

Challenge 5: Physical Limitations

If you have physical limitations, like joint pain or neuropathy, exercise can feel daunting. But that doesn't mean you can't be active.

Strategies to Work Around Limitations

1. Choose Low-Impact Activities: Swimming, cycling, and yoga are great options for people with joint pain or mobility issues.

2. Modify Exercises: If an exercise is too difficult, modify it to suit your abilities. For example, do wall push-ups instead of regular push-ups.

3. Work with a Professional: A physical therapist or certified personal trainer can help you create a safe and effective workout plan.

Challenge 6: Lack of Support

it's hard to stay motivated when you don't have support from the people around you.

Strategies to Build a Support System

1. Communicate Your Goals: Let your family and friends know why exercise is important to you and how they can support you.

2. Find a Workout Buddy: Exercising with a friend can make it more fun and keep you accountable.

3. Join a Community: Look for local or online groups for people with diabetes or fitness enthusiasts.

Share your progress on social media to connect with others and stay motivated.

Challenge 7: Plateaus

At some point, you might hit a plateau where you stop seeing progress. It's frustrating, but it's also a normal part of the fitness journey.

Strategies to Break Through Plateaus

1. Change Your Routine: If you've been doing the same workout for weeks, try something new to challenge your body.

2. Increase Intensity: Add more resistance, speed, or duration to your workouts.

3. Reassess Your Goals: Are your goals still realistic? Do they need to be adjusted?

Chapter 6

Nutrition and Exercise—The Dynamic Duo

You can't out-exercise a bad diet. No matter how many miles you run or how many weights you lift, if your nutrition isn't on point, you're fighting an uphill battle. This is especially true when you're managing diabetes.

Exercise and nutrition are like peanut butter and jelly—they're great on their own, but together, they're unstoppable. In this chapter, we're diving deep into how to fuel your body for exercise, manage your blood sugar, and make smart food choices that support your fitness goals.

Why Nutrition Matters

When you have diabetes, what you eat directly impacts your blood sugar levels. Add exercise into the mix, and it becomes even more important to pay attention to your nutrition.

Exercise increases your body's demand for glucose, which can lower your blood sugar levels. But if you don't fuel properly, you could end up with low blood sugar (hypoglycemia) or feel sluggish and unmotivated. On the flip side, eating the wrong foods can cause your blood sugar to spike, undoing all the hard work you put into your workout.

Pre-Workout Nutrition: Fueling Up

What you eat before a workout can make or break your performance. The goal is to provide your body with enough energy to get through your exercise without causing a blood sugar spike or crash.

What to Eat Before a Workout

1. Complex Carbs: These provide a steady source of energy. Think whole grains, fruits, and vegetables.

2. Protein: Helps stabilize blood sugar and supports muscle repair. Examples include Greek yogurt, eggs, or a handful of nuts.

3. Healthy Fats: Provide long-lasting energy. Avocado, nut butter, or a small handful of seeds are great options.

Eat your pre-workout snack 30-60 minutes before exercising to give your body time to digest.

During-Workout Nutrition: Staying Powered Up

For most people, a quick workout doesn't require mid-exercise snacks. But if you're doing a long or intense session, you might need a little boost to keep your energy levels stable.

What to Eat During a Workout

1. Fast-Acting Carbs: If your blood sugar drops, reach for something that can raise it quickly, like glucose tablets, fruit juice, or a small piece of candy.

2. Hydration: Drink water or a sugar-free sports drink to stay hydrated.

If you're exercising for more than an hour, consider having a small snack, like a piece of fruit or a granola bar, to keep your energy up.

Post-Workout Nutrition: Recovery and Repair

After a workout, your body needs nutrients to recover and rebuild. This is especially important for people with diabetes, as exercise can lower blood sugar levels for several hours afterward.

What to Eat After a Workout

1. Protein: Helps repair and build muscle. Examples include chicken, fish, tofu, or a protein shake.

2. Complex Carbs: Replenish glycogen stores and stabilize blood sugar. Think quinoa, sweet potatoes, or whole-grain bread.

3. Healthy Fats: Support overall recovery. Avocado, olive oil, or a handful of nuts are great options.

Aim to eat within 30-60 minutes after your workout to maximize recovery.

Managing Blood Sugar Around Exercise

Exercise can have a big impact on your blood sugar levels, so it's important to monitor them closely and make adjustments as needed.

Tips for Managing Blood Sugar

1. Check Before and After: Always check your blood sugar before and after exercise to see how your body responds.

2. Adjust Your Meals: If you know you're going to exercise, you might need to adjust your meals or snacks to prevent lows or highs.

3. Carry Snacks: Keep fast-acting carbs nearby in case your blood sugar drops during your workout.

The Role of Hydration

Staying hydrated is crucial for everyone, but it's especially important when you have diabetes.

Dehydration can affect your blood sugar levels and make it harder for your body to regulate temperature during exercise.

Tips for Staying Hydrated

1. Drink Water Throughout the Day: Don't wait until you're thirsty to drink water.

2. Monitor Your Urine: If it's pale yellow, you're hydrated. If it's dark, drink more water.

3. Avoid Sugary Drinks: Stick to water or sugar-free beverages to avoid blood sugar spikes.

If you're doing a long or intense workout, consider a sports drink with electrolytes to replace what you lose through sweat.

Making Smart Food Choices

When you have diabetes, every meal and snack is an opportunity to support your health. Here are some tips for making smart food choices:

1. Focus on Whole Foods: Choose foods that are as close to their natural state as possible, like fruits, vegetables, lean proteins, and whole grains.

2. Limit Processed Foods: These are often high in sugar, salt, and unhealthy fats, which can wreak havoc on your blood sugar.

3. Read Labels: Pay attention to serving sizes, carb counts, and added sugars.

Chapter 7

Staying Motivated for the Long Haul

Starting a fitness routine is one thing, but sticking with it? That's where the real challenge lies. Life gets busy. Motivation wanes. And sometimes, it feels easier to just hit the snooze button and skip your workout. But here's the thing: staying motivated isn't about willpower or discipline. It's about creating habits, setting yourself up for success, and finding joy in the process.

Why Motivation Fades (And What to Do About It)

Motivation is like a fire—it burns bright at first, but without fuel, it eventually dies out. The key to staying motivated is to keep adding fuel to the fire.

Here are some common reasons why motivation fades and how to reignite it:

1. Lack of Progress: If you're not seeing results, it's easy to get discouraged.

- Solution: Focus on small wins and non-scale victories, like feeling more energized or sleeping better.

2. Boredom: Doing the same workout over and over can get monotonous.

- Solution: Mix it up! Try new activities, join a class, or set a fun challenge.

3. Burnout: Pushing yourself too hard can lead to exhaustion and burnout.

- Solution: Take rest days, listen to your body, and prioritize recovery.

Building Habits That Stick

Motivation might get you started, but habits are what keep you going. The good news? Building habits doesn't have to be complicated.

Tips for Building Habits

1. Start Small: Focus on one small change at a time, like walking 10 minutes a day.

2. Be Consistent: Do your new habit at the same time every day to make it stick.

3. Stack Habits: Pair your new habit with something you already do, like doing squats while you brush your teeth.

Use a habit tracker to keep yourself accountable and celebrate your progress.

Finding Your Why

When the going gets tough, your "why" is what will keep you going. Why did you start this journey in the first place? What's your bigger purpose?

How to Find Your Why

1. Reflect on Your Goals: What do you want to achieve? How will it improve your life?

2. Think About Your Loved Ones: How will your health impact your ability to spend time with them?

3. Visualize Your Future Self: What kind of person do you want to be in 5, 10, or 20 years?

Setting Realistic Goals

Setting goals is important, but they need to be realistic and achievable. Otherwise, you're setting yourself up for disappointment.

Tips for Setting Goals

1. Be Specific: Instead of saying, "I want to get fit," say, "I want to walk 30 minutes a day, 5 days a week."

2. Break It Down: Divide your big goal into smaller, more manageable steps.

3. Celebrate Progress: Acknowledge and celebrate every small win along the way.

Use the SMART framework—Specific, Measurable, Achievable, Relevant, and Time-bound—to set effective goals.

Staying Accountable

Accountability is a powerful motivator. When you know someone is counting on you, you're more likely to follow through.

Tips for Staying Accountable

1. Find a Workout Buddy: Exercising with a friend can make it more fun and keep you on track.

2. Join a Community: Look for local or online groups for people with similar goals.

3. Share Your Progress: Post about your workouts on social media or keep a journal to track your progress.

Making It Fun

if you're not having fun, you're not going to stick with it. The key to long-term success is finding activities you genuinely enjoy.

Tips for Making Exercise Fun

1. Try New Activities: Experiment with different types of exercise until you find something you love.

2. Incorporate Play: Turn your workout into a game or challenge.

3. Listen to Music or Podcasts: Create a workout playlist or listen to your favorite podcast to make the time fly by.

If you're a social person, try group fitness classes or team sports.

Dealing with Setbacks

Setbacks are a normal part of any journey, but they don't have to derail your progress. The key is to learn from them and keep moving forward.

Tips for Dealing with Setbacks

1. Be Kind to Yourself: Don't beat yourself up over a missed workout or a bad day.

2. Reflect and Adjust: What caused the setback? How can you prevent it from happening again?

3. Get Back on Track: Focus on what you can do today to get back on track.

Celebrating Your Wins

Celebrating your wins—big and small—is crucial for staying motivated. It reminds you of how far you've come and keeps you excited about the journey ahead.

Chapter 8

Building a Support System That Works

You don't have to do this alone. Managing diabetes and staying fit is a team effort, and having the right support system can make all the difference. Whether it's friends, family, or a community of like-minded individuals, the people around you can provide encouragement, accountability, and even a little tough love when you need it.

Why Support Matters

When you're trying to make lifestyle changes, having a support system can be the difference between success and failure. Here's why:

1. Accountability: When someone is counting on you, you're more likely to follow through.

2. Encouragement: A little encouragement can go a long way, especially on tough days.

3. Shared Knowledge: Your support system can offer tips, advice, and resources you might not have thought of.

Communicating Your Needs

The first step in building a support system is communicating your needs. people can't support you if they don't know what you need.

Tips for Communicating Your Needs

1. Be Honest: Share your goals, challenges, and what kind of support you're looking for.

2. Be Specific: Instead of saying, "I need support," say, "I'd love it if you could join me for a walk after dinner."

3. Express Gratitude: Let people know how much their support means to you.

Use "I" statements to express your needs without sounding accusatory. For example, "I feel more motivated when we exercise together."

Finding Your Tribe

Your support system doesn't have to be limited to friends and family. There are countless communities—both online and offline—where you can find like-minded individuals who share your goals.

Tips for Finding Your Tribe

1. Join a Support Group: Look for local or online groups for people with diabetes or fitness enthusiasts.

2. Take a Class: Group fitness classes are a great way to meet people who share your interests.

3. Use Social Media: Follow influencers, join Facebook groups, or participate in online challenges.

Don't be afraid to put yourself out there. The more you engage, the more connections you'll make.

Creating a Supportive Environment

Your environment plays a huge role in your success. If you're surrounded by junk food and negativity, it's going to be a lot harder to stay on track.

Tips for Creating a Supportive Environment

1. Stock Healthy Foods: Fill your kitchen with nutritious options that support your goals.

2. Set Boundaries: Let people know what behaviors are helpful and what's not.

3. Create a Workout Space: Even if it's just a corner of your living room, having a dedicated space can make it easier to stick with your routine.

Dealing with Unsupportive People

Not everyone is going to be supportive, and that's okay. The key is to focus on the people who are and not let the naysayers bring you down.

Tips for Dealing with Unsupportive People

1. Set Boundaries: Let people know what kind of behavior is acceptable and what's not.

2. Focus on the Positive: Surround yourself with people who uplift and encourage you.

3. Let It Go: Don't waste your energy trying to change someone who's not willing to support you.

Remember, their lack of support says more about them than it does about you.

Chapter 9

Tracking Progress and Staying Accountable

Staying on track with your fitness and diabetes management goals isn't just about motivation or willpower. It's about having a system in place to track your progress, celebrate your wins, and hold yourself accountable. Without a clear way to measure how far you've come, it's easy to lose sight of your goals or feel like you're spinning your wheels.

Why Tracking Progress Matters

When you're managing diabetes and working on your fitness, tracking your progress is like having a roadmap. It shows you where you've been, where you're going, and how far you've come.

Here's why tracking matters:

1. It Keeps You Honest: When you track your progress, there's no room for guesswork. You know exactly what you've accomplished and where you need to improve.

2. It Boosts Motivation: Seeing your progress—even small wins—can give you the motivation to keep going.

3. It Helps You Adjust: If something isn't working, tracking your progress can help you identify the problem and make changes.

What to Track

Tracking your progress doesn't have to be complicated. The key is to focus on the metrics that matter most to your goals.

1. Blood Sugar Levels

Tracking your blood sugar is essential for managing diabetes. It helps you understand how your body responds to different foods, activities, and medications.

- How to Track: Use a blood glucose monitor or a continuous glucose monitor (CGM) to check your levels regularly.

- What to Look For: Pay attention to patterns and trends, like how your blood sugar responds to exercise or certain foods.

Keep a log of your blood sugar levels, including the time of day, what you ate, and any exercise you did.

2. Workouts

Tracking your workouts helps you stay consistent and see progress over time.

- How to Track: Use a workout journal, app, or wearable device to log your exercises, duration, and intensity.

- What to Look For: Focus on improvements, like running faster, lifting heavier weights, or feeling less fatigued.

Set specific goals for your workouts, like increasing your steps or adding more reps, and track your progress toward those goals.

3. Nutrition

Tracking what you eat can help you make smarter food choices and manage your blood sugar levels.

- How to Track: Use a food diary, app, or even photos to log your meals and snacks.

- What to Look For: Pay attention to how different foods affect your energy, mood, and blood sugar levels.

Focus on balance rather than perfection. Aim for a mix of protein, carbs, and healthy fats at each meal.

How to Stay Accountable

Accountability is the secret sauce to staying on track. When you know someone is counting on you, you're more likely to follow through.

Tips for Staying Accountable

1. Find a Workout Buddy: Exercising with a friend can make it more fun and keep you on track.

2. Join a Community: Look for local or online groups for people with similar goals.

3. Share Your Progress: Post about your workouts on social media or keep a journal to track your progress.

Celebrating Your Wins

Celebrating your wins—big and small—is crucial for staying motivated. It reminds you of how far you've come and keeps you excited about the journey ahead.

Tips for Celebrating Wins

1. Acknowledge Your Progress: Take a moment to reflect on what you've accomplished.

2. Reward Yourself: Treat yourself to something you enjoy, like a new workout outfit or a relaxing massage.

3. Share Your Success: Celebrate with friends, family, or your support community.

Keep a journal or scrapbook to document your progress and celebrate your wins.

Dealing with Setbacks

Setbacks are a normal part of any journey, but they don't have to derail your progress. The key is to learn from them and keep moving forward.

Tips for Dealing with Setbacks

1. Be Kind to Yourself: Don't beat yourself up over a missed workout or a bad day.

2. Reflect and Adjust: What caused the setback? How can you prevent it from happening again?

3. Get Back on Track: Focus on what you can do today to get back on track.

Chapter 10

Long-Term Success—Making Fitness a Lifestyle

Anyone can start a fitness routine. The hard part is sticking with it for the long haul. Life gets busy, motivation wanes, and old habits creep back in. But here's the thing: fitness isn't a sprint; it's a marathon. It's not about quick fixes or temporary changes. It's about creating a lifestyle that supports your health and well-being for years to come.

Why Long-Term Success Matters

When it comes to managing diabetes and staying fit, consistency is key. Short-term changes might give you quick results, but they're not sustainable. Long-term success is about creating habits and routines that become second nature.

Here's why long-term success matters:

1. It's Sustainable: Long-term changes are easier to maintain because they become part of your daily life.

2. It's Healthier: Consistent exercise and healthy eating have long-term benefits for your physical and mental health.

3. It's Empowering: When you make fitness a lifestyle, you're in control of your health and well-being.

Building Habits That Stick

The key to long-term success is building habits that stick. Habits are automatic behaviors that require little to no thought or effort. The more habits you build, the easier it becomes to stay on track.

Tips for Building Habits

1. Start Small: Focus on one small change at a time, like walking 10 minutes a day.

2. Be Consistent: Do your new habit at the same time every day to make it stick.

3. Stack Habits: Pair your new habit with something you already do, like doing squats while you brush your teeth.

Use a habit tracker to keep yourself accountable and celebrate your progress.

Overcoming Obstacles

Life is full of obstacles, but they don't have to derail your progress. The key is to anticipate challenges and have a plan in place to overcome them.

Common Obstacles and How to Overcome Them

1. Lack of Time: Break your workouts into smaller chunks or multitask by exercising while watching TV.

2. Low Motivation: Find activities you enjoy and set small, achievable goals to keep yourself motivated.

3. Setbacks: Don't beat yourself up over a missed workout or a bad day. Focus on what you can do today to get back on track.

Creating a Supportive Environment

Your environment plays a huge role in your success. If you're surrounded by junk food and negativity, it's going to be a lot harder to stay on track.

Tips for Creating a Supportive Environment

1. Stock Healthy Foods: Fill your kitchen with nutritious options that support your goals.

2. Set Boundaries: Let people know what behaviors are helpful and what's not.

3. Create a Workout Space: Even if it's just a corner of your living room, having a dedicated space can make it easier to stick with your routine.

Staying Accountable

Accountability is the secret sauce to staying on track. When you know someone is counting on you, you're more likely to follow through.

Tips for Staying Accountable

1. Find a Workout Buddy: Exercising with a friend can make it more fun and keep you on track.

2. Join a Community: Look for local or online groups for people with similar goals.

3. Share Your Progress: Post about your workouts on social media or keep a journal to track your progress.

Printed in Dunstable, United Kingdom